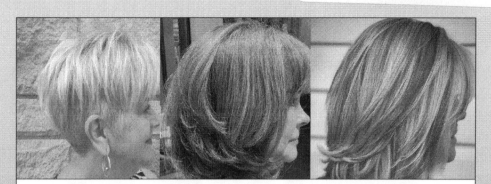

80 Best Modern Hairstyles and Haircuts for Women over 50 In 2023

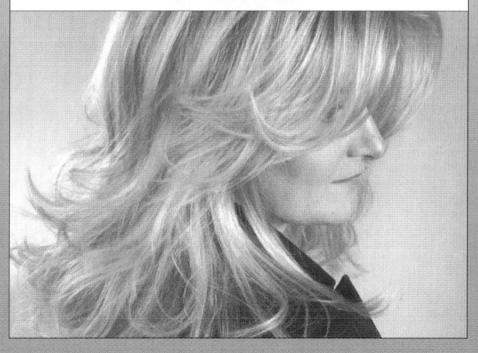

Haircuts for Women Over 50 In 2023

Explore 80 outstanding hairstyle options to update your look, including timeless classics like bobs, layered cuts, pixie cuts, and gentle waves. Choose a contemporary and polished hairdo for 2023 that suits your particular style.

MARGARET R. SAXTON

Table of Contents

Blunt Nape-Length Bob

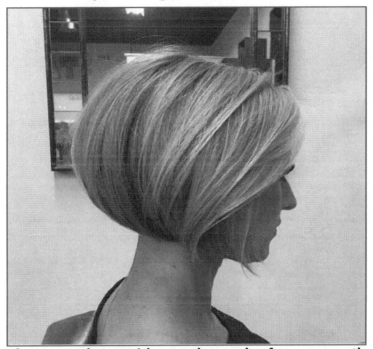

There are always girls out there who favour smooth haircuts, even when dishevelled hair is quite popular. If you want a precise and clean cut for thick, straight hair, try this stylish bob.

These images can serve as inspiration, then. Consider picking a hairdo that will highlight your personality's defining characteristics and represent your character. Make sure everyone knows how pleasant, joyful, and youthful you still are.

Layered Bronde Bob Over 50

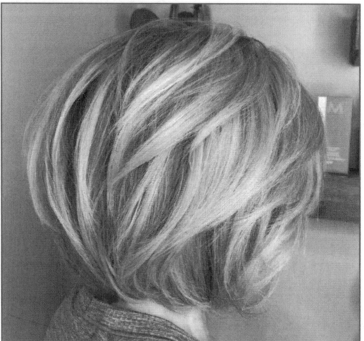

Combine a multi-toned hue with jagged layers and a cropped bob. The bob has a pixie-cut impression because to the texture from the layers, yet you may still enjoy collarbone-length hair.

Smart Ultra-Short Bob

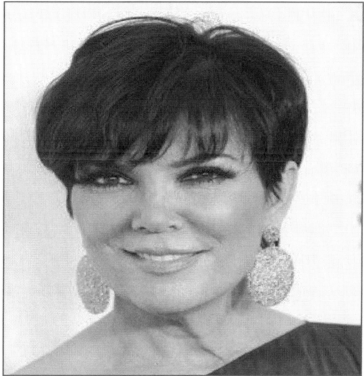

Oval faces look fantastic with really short bobs that have volume at the top and graduated edges. Black hair with faint chocolate feathers is perfect for highlighting the dark brown eyes.

Roundbrush Bob

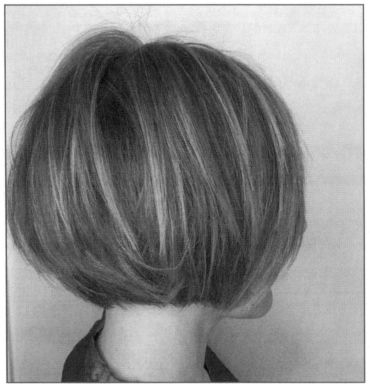

There are short women's haircuts that might assist soften an angular face. With a fast round-brushing session, the layers in this bob would soften into smooth, curving lines that would frame your face.

Sassy Silver Gray Pixie

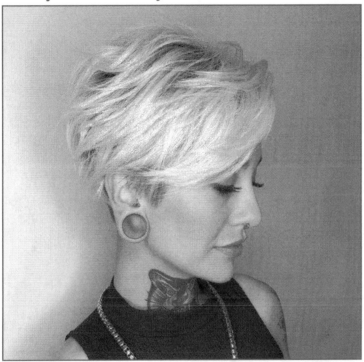

It's astonishing how attractive one of every woman's worst worries - Gray hairs - may look in trendy sassy haircuts. A trendy pixie with broken outlines is a great option!

Medium Strawberry Blonde Hairstyle with Swoopy Layers

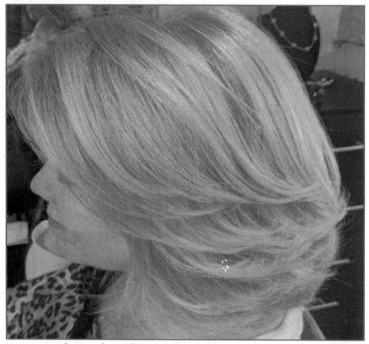

You can have beach-worthy hair every day with long, angled layers. Side bangs will always blend nicely with this style. If you need a colour refresh, choose a subtle strawberry blonde tint!

Classic Blonde Bob

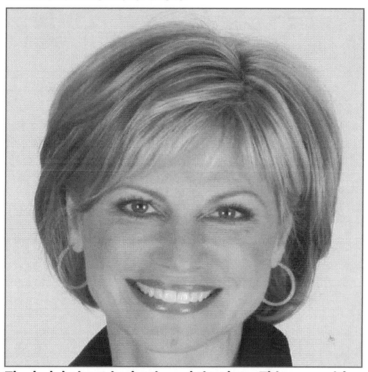

The bob haircut is classic and timeless. This one, with a side part and precise grading for the tresses framing the face, is ideal for ladies over 50 with fine straight hair.

Lisa Rinna Like

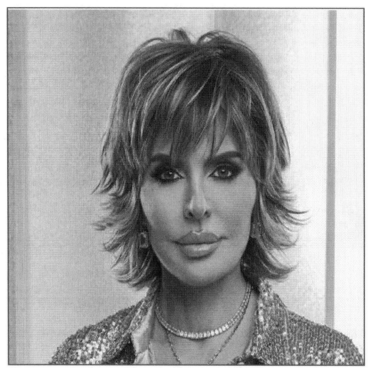

If you desire this trademark haircut, ask your hairdresser for a medium-thick hair cut with layering below the mid-ear point. Brown highlights will add dimension and accentuate the texture of dark brown hair.

Flipped Blonde Lob

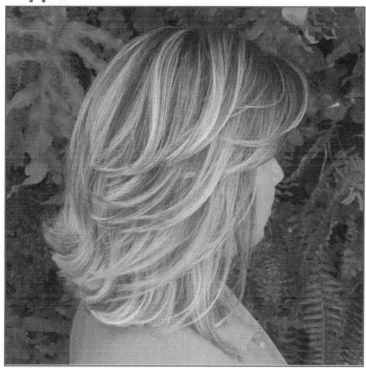

The openness and clean lines of this stunning classic hairdo provide a very respectable vibe. And the extensive layering along the mid-ear area merely adds to the liveliness and modernity.

Sassy and Sexy Pixie

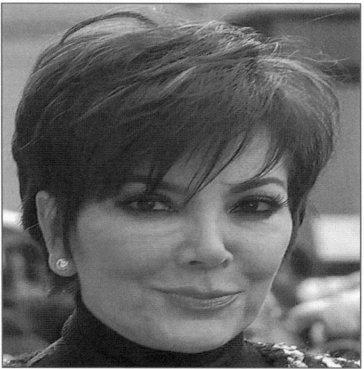

This raven pixie with a feathery finish is impossible to resist. It seems modern and a touch sassy, which is exactly what is in demand for good-looking ladies over 50 with class and style in their veins.

Mid-Length Hairstyle with Body-Building Layers

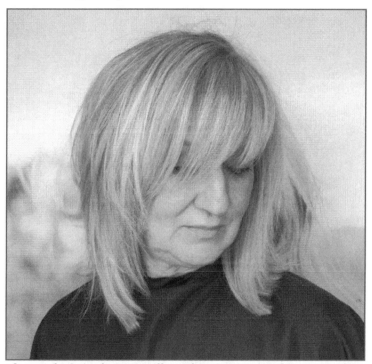

If your hair isn't naturally voluminous, go for a cut that adds volume with clever layers. Pair them with bangs, and all you'll need to do for style is teasing the roots, tousling the lengths, and spritzing with hairspray. Hairstyles for women over 50 should be simple and natural-looking.

MARGARET R. SAXTON

Blonde Slanted Bob with Layers

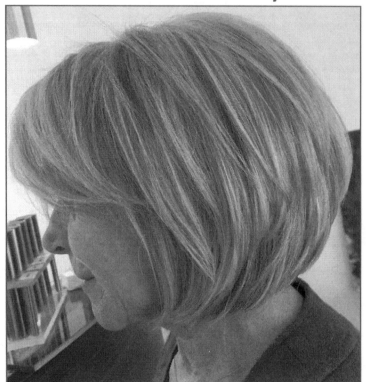

With the aid of the dynamic combo of layers and highlights, you can effortlessly amp up hairstyles for women over 50. The slanted bob is a beautiful design that works well with both straight and curly hair.

Cute Layered Gray Pixie

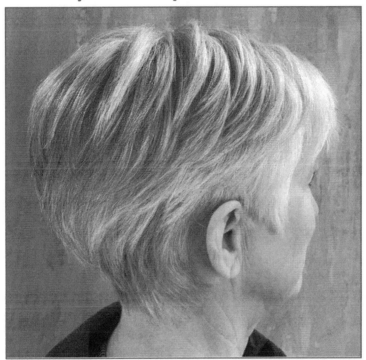

Do you wear glasses all the time? A layered pixie design is ideal for complementing your favorite frames. The crop with V-cut layers provides the necessary structure for your face shape, and adding charming side bangs will complement your spectacles.

Short Feathered Gray Hairstyle

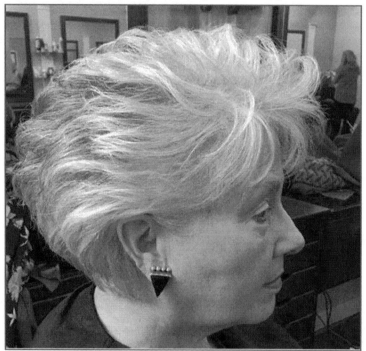

It's always fun to channel past decades in a modern way in today's popular hairstyles. With this bob cut, you'll be bringing back the '80s through short, feathery layers and teased roots. Don't be afraid to show off your grey hair with this dramatic style!

Long Bombshell Red Locks

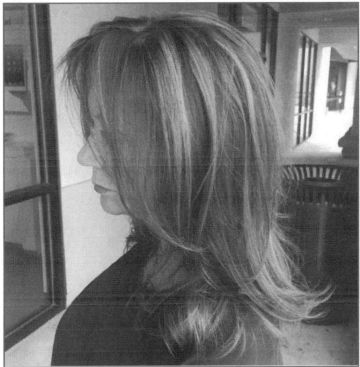

This look is long and vibrant, proving that over 50 haircuts and styles don't have to be dull - all it takes is a sassy attitude to pull off! A crimson foundation with blonde accents will definitely warm up your skin!

MARGARET R. SAXTON

20

Light Copper Bob with Blonde Highlights

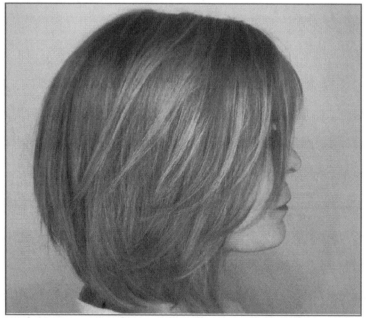

Updating your colon and even experimenting with a new shade is a terrific way to keep your style appearing young and fresh. Copper tones peppered with tiny blonde highlights distributed throughout your hair create a look that you may have worn in your twenties.

Buttery Blonde Mid-Length Hair

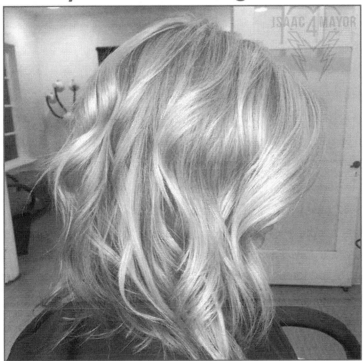

Blonde is a common hue for older women's hairstyles that helps to disguise grey hair: grey roots react better to bleach than colour, and re-growth is less obvious against a lighter shade. This gorgeous, buttery golden mane would look wonderful at any age, but it's best reserved for very healthy hair.

MARGARET R. SAXTON

Long Feathered Pixie with Sideburns

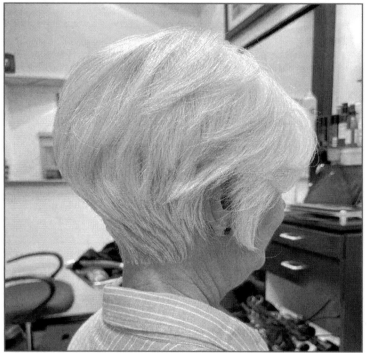

Think sideburns are only for men? Think again. Think again, since this sassy spin on the traditional pixie cut might become your new go-to look. Women's hairstyles frequently take characteristics from men's trends, and complementing them with feminine accents, such as voluminous feathery layers, makes the final appearance even more elegant.

MARGARET R. SAXTON

Medium Cut with Feathered Layers

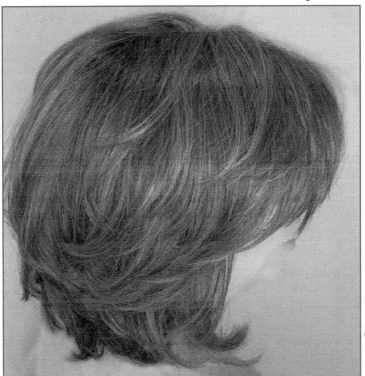

The greatest haircuts for women over 50 are those that do a good job of accentuating the facial traits you like and masking the ones you don't. If you add swoopy peek-a-boo bangs to a traditional medium hairstyle with layers, you'll seem fashionable and younger - which never hurts!

MARGARET R. SAXTON

Warm and Wavy Lob

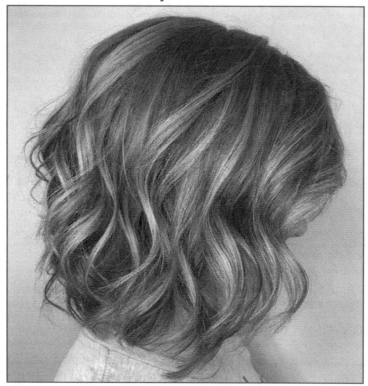

If you're looking for trendy hairstyles for women over 50, try this hairdo, which has randomly placed, alternating curls. It retains its professional appearance owing to a sleek, side-swept bang. The warm brown colour also exudes young vitality.

Shoulder-Grazing Wispy Cut

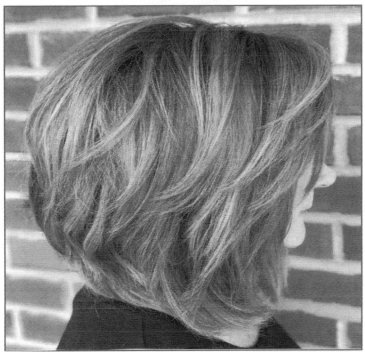

If you have fine hair, make sure you select a style that complements rather than contrasts your texture. Choosing a wispy, layered cut will add movement to otherwise straight and lifeless strands.

Mid-Length Hairstyle with Overlapping Layers

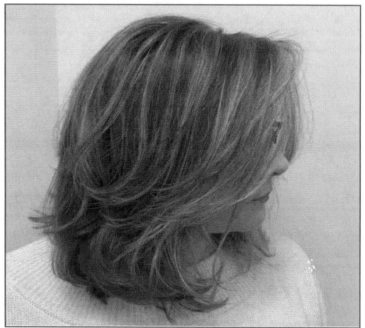

When it comes to mid-length styles, it's critical to do everything possible to bring movement and flow to your cut. Overlapping layers provide a lovely wave effect. Not to add that this hairstyle is simple to style, so you won't waste much time in front of the mirror.

Short Layered Ash Blonde Hairstyle

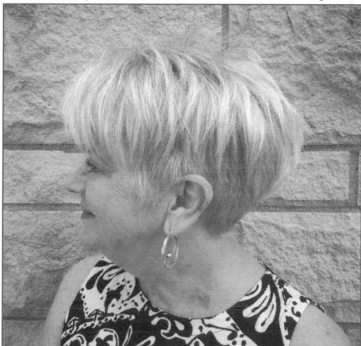

Layers may look just as well in shorter female hairstyles as they do in longer ones, but you must understand how to make the layers work for your specific hair structure. Smooth layers in a long pixie on straight hair structure the cut and add flawless smoothness and evenness to the finished look.

Neat Layered Two-Tone Bob

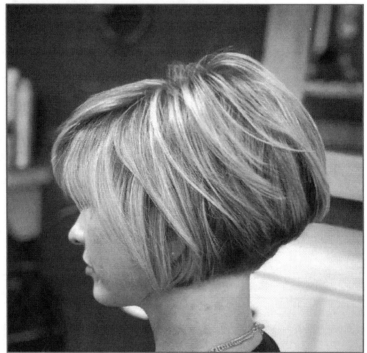

When it comes to picking a haircut for your 50s, some people believe that prim and polished is the way to go. Instead of jagged or razored layers, keep your trimmed bob looking smooth. Because this haircut is so clean-cut, add some personality to it with a sophisticated balayage.

MARGARET R. SAXTON

Long Feathered Walnut Brown Pixie

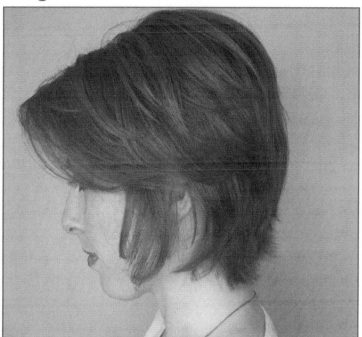

Try a short bob or a long, feathery pixie cut if you like shorter hair. The feathery layers on top and the tapering neck make this a classic haircut for a confident older woman.

Over 50 Medium Curly Hairstyle with Bangs

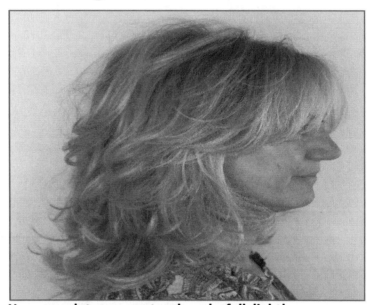

You may let your natural curls fall lightly over your shoulders with medium length hair. Play experiment with different blond tones to bring the look together and make the curls more dimensional. For a classic 1970s shag look, pair your ringlets with a point cut fringe.

Medium Feathered Golden Bronde Cut

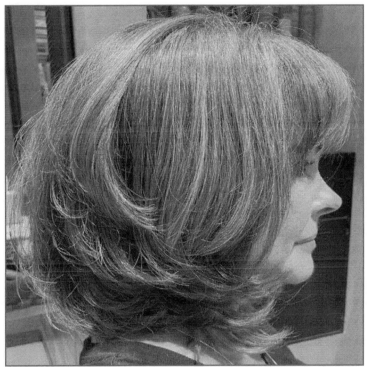

If you're ready to say goodbye to lengthy hairstyles that don't highlight your greatest facial features, this medium-length bronde shag will bring out all the charms you've been concealing. The elegant hairstyle is separated in the center and has a lot of feathery layers, giving it a young look that's super-easy to maintain.

MARGARET R. SAXTON

Pixie Bob with Stacked Layers in the Back

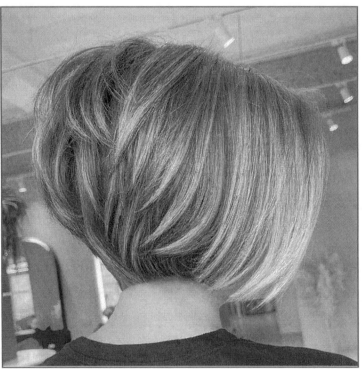

Over-50 females' hairstyles frequently blend natural gray into the color job to make it seem lovely and meaningful. With this style, you can show off your natural color by blending greys with delicate highlights. Shorten the layers in the back for a natural lift.

MARGARET R. SAXTON

Delicate Wavy Golden Blonde Bob

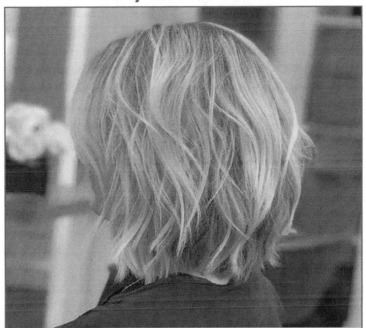

Bobs are one of our top hairstyles for women over 50. Allow your golden blonde waves to flow into a natural pattern to make the most of them. Part your bangs in the center or sweep them to one side for an ultra-feminine look that frames your face perfectly.

Short Crop with Side Bangs

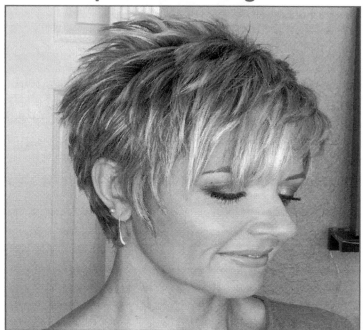

Short hairstyles for women over 50 are popular for a reason: they are simple to style and have a unique flair. Consider mixing the cropped-short back and longer bangs in your favorite short haircut, as seen in this lovely pixie.

Short-to-Medium Feathered Cut

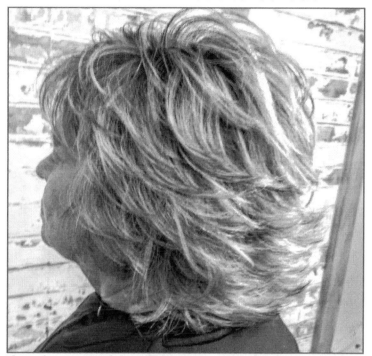

If you're a round-faced over-50 woman, you confront a unique set of challenges: how to seem younger, healthier, and smaller. A short-to-medium feathery cut might help you attain the look. A large face may be narrowed down with side-swept bangs and layers that fall in front of the ears.

MARGARET R. SAXTON

Shoulder Length Hairstyle with Flicked Out Ends

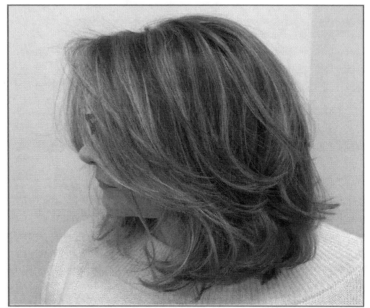

There is no reason to have an unnecessarily intricate hairstyle. At your age, you should strive for healthy hair with a good finish. The way the ends of this hairstyle have been stacked and turned out is stunning. It is appropriate for both everyday use and more formal settings.

Mid-Length Hairdo with Bangs

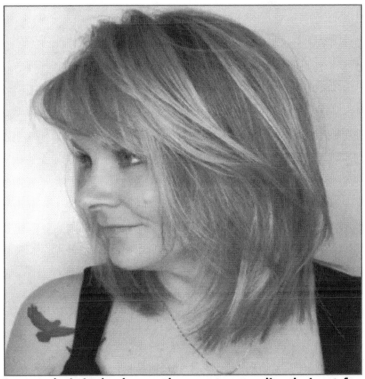

Longer hair isn't always the most appealing haircut for women over 50, especially if your locks are thin. If you still want long hairstyles and want to go with something that will look well on your fine hair, the appropriate layering will make your medium to long hairstyle stand out.

MARGARET R. SAXTON

Straight Blonde Bob with Bangs

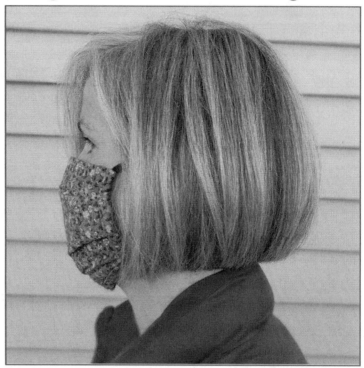

A bob is a timeless style that suits people of all ages. It all comes down to picking the correct form, length, and color to complement your characteristics. Adding a fringe and delicate highlights around your face is a fantastic experiment.

Medium Style with Blonde Highlights

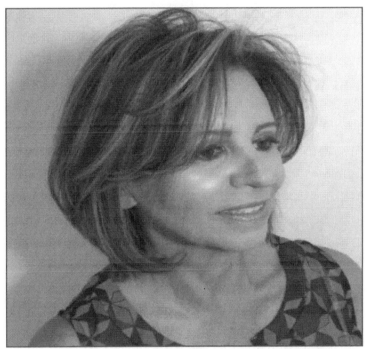

Many hairstyles for women over 50 are cropped, but there are also many beautiful medium and long choices. If you want some length but don't want Rapunzel-like strands, anything that touches around the shoulders is preferable.

Short Bright Razored Pixie Over 50

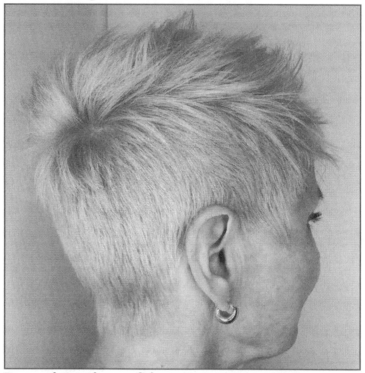

Do you have the confidence to sport a gorgeous super-short pixie cut on your fine hair? If you're a woman over the age of 50, you should! Short haircuts are one of the most effective methods for a lady to appear younger. The spiky crown part attracts attention upward, elevating and somewhat elongating the face.

Bold and Spiky Pixie

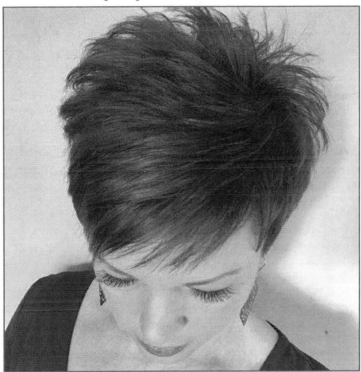

You may bring out your innate beauty by pairing a bright color with a simple cut. For example, the spiky pixie appears complex but is surprisingly simple to style. The sassy spikes may be brushed forward and groomed with wax. Different hair color variations can provide more complexity to the cut.

MARGARET R. SAXTON

Medium Feathered Beige Blonde Cut

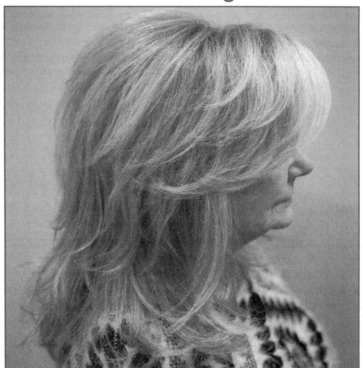

Side-swept feathered bangs and a slight lift in the crown section can make haircuts for women over 50 more youthful and carefree. The light beige color does a wonderful job of hiding those pesky grays. The length of the hair shown in this picture is just right, hitting slightly below the shoulders.

MARGARET R. SAXTON

Highlights and Lowlights in Medium Length Cut

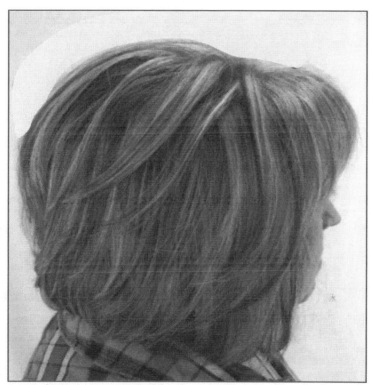

Long hair is not suitable for everyone. But it doesn't mean you have to keep it incredibly short. This is the ideal medium-length cut for richness and depth. A perfect 10 in hairstyles for elderly ladies is soft layers with light and dark strands intermingled throughout.

MARGARET R. SAXTON

Crisp Wispy Light Blonde Bob

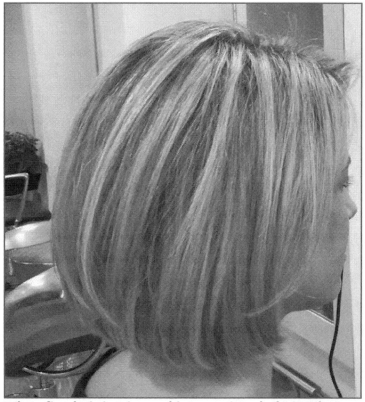

When fine hair is trimmed into a wispy bob, it takes on a whole new dimension. To keep the illusion of fullness, alternate the portion from one side to the other and tousle the top.

Medium Piece-y Cut for Thick Hair

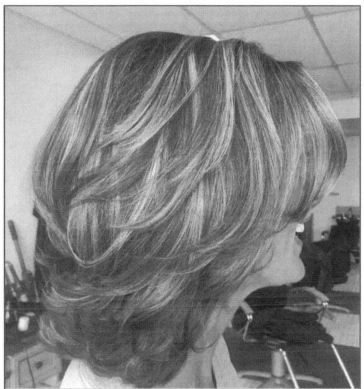

Medium-length hairstyles with piece-y layers are ideal for women over 50 with thick hair. The longish "peek-a-boo" bangs serve to conceal those pesky wrinkles around the eyes and brow, and the silver-white highlights over an ash brown foundation provide a fashionable and current touch.

MARGARET R. SAXTON

46

Medium Voluminous Straight Blonde Hair

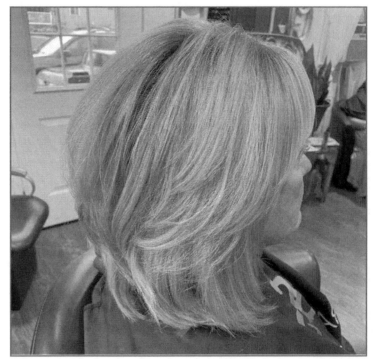

Who says haircuts for those over 50 have to be dull and drab? Light and airy layered shags add a youthful vitality to your face, making you look 10 years younger. Wispy bangs strategically placed might conceal places you don't want to draw attention to.

Medium Straight Blowout Hairstyle

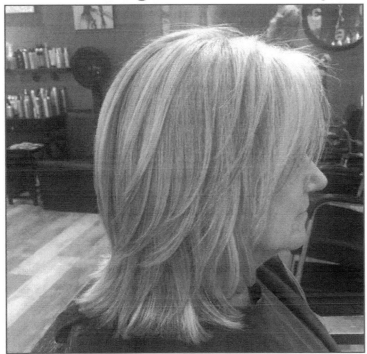

Long, thin hair looks best when cut into a lob, with the bulk of the strands skirting the shoulders. Ask your hairdresser create lengthy layers that hit an inch or two over the edge of your cut to provide the illusion of lift. Because there's nothing short to provide texture to the top, keep everything glossy and sleek by going straight.

MARGARET R. SAXTON

48

Fun Silver Pixie with Long Razored Layers

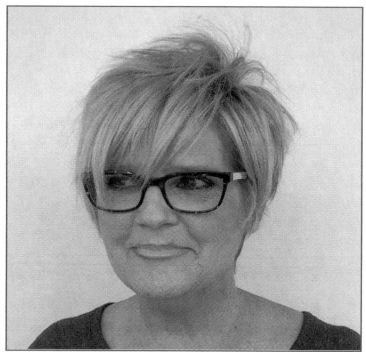

Making the front layers and bangs into one is a particularly interesting way to personalize a pixie cut. Many women's haircuts separate bangs from the rest of the style, but when the entire appearance is razored, certain forward-facing strands can generate bangs on their own. Silver hair coloring is a fashionable remedy for graying hair.

MARGARET R. SAXTON

Over 50 Feathered Blonde Pixie Bob

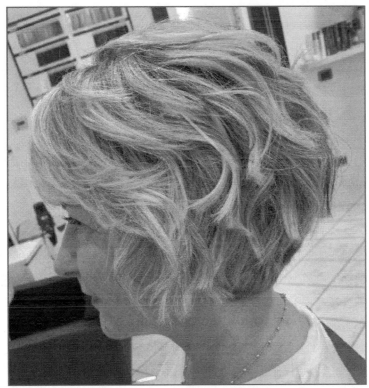

While a pixie is a shorter haircut, the layers themselves may be as long as you choose. Straightening hair gives the appearance of longer locks, but maintaining it piecey lets each strand stand out. Apply a dry oil spray on the form to provide gloss, hold, and definition.

MARGARET R. SAXTON

50

Short-to-Medium Feathered Voluminous Cut

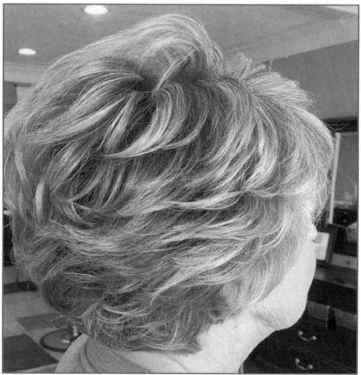

Older ladies who wish to seem young and energetic must choose haircuts that suit them. Short to medium haircuts are often favored since they minimize the troublesome jaw line and chin regions. Maintaining the crown portion feathered gives much-needed height and pizzazz.

MARGARET R. SAXTON

Cute Feathered Brown Pixie Over 50

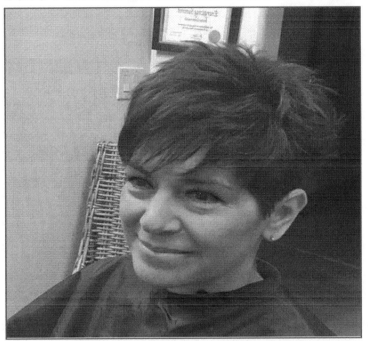

Many hairstyles for older women don't require any heat at all, especially if you have amazing natural texture! Feathered layers allow thicker, wavy, or curly hair to be chopped short without seeming too helmet-like. Add some texturizing paste and style to your liking.

MARGARET R. SAXTON

Over 50 Messy Pixie Bob Hairstyle

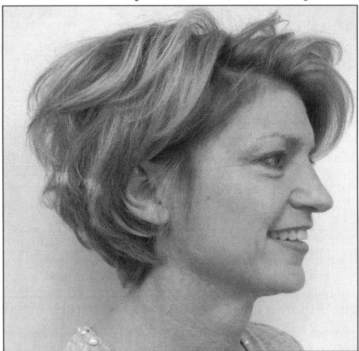

Not all short hairstyles are intended to be tidy and polished. With this messy long pixie, you may embrace the fashionable undone appearance. The staggered layers give the style movement, and the uneven component emphasizes the 'do's intrinsic feeling of exquisite imperfection. This cut is ideal for ladies with long faces since the waves and layers will balance out the length of your face.

MARGARET R. SAXTON

Blonde Pixie

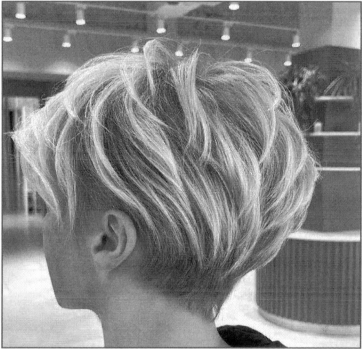

Pixie cuts are popular among middle-aged ladies for good reason! The tapered profile maintains the appearance of length in the front and at the top while eliminating the daily care required by longer hair. When wearing this style, keep the hair around the nape of the neck clean to retain a polished appearance.

Voluminous Nape-Length Tapered Cut

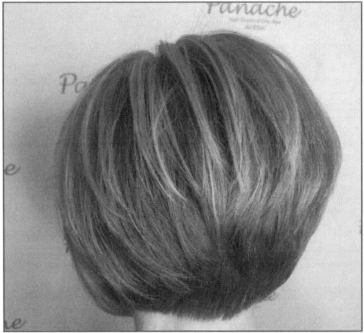

Try a new take on the classic bob haircut, which has been popular for many generations. With piece-y layers, add some lift to the crown. The honey golden tones with light blonde highlights provide the tapered cut a refined, professional appearance without seeming "too old."

MARGARET R. SAXTON

Neck-Length Hairstyle with Razored Layers

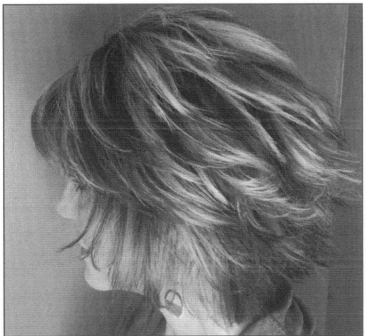

Feathered hairstyles for thin hair for ladies over 50 are ideal for plumping up dull and worn locks. By cutting it short, you may give volume and lift to areas of thinning hair. Straight locks and bronde tones frame the face and highlight your attributes.

MARGARET R. SAXTON

56

Cute Razored Metallic Bronde Cut for Medium Hair

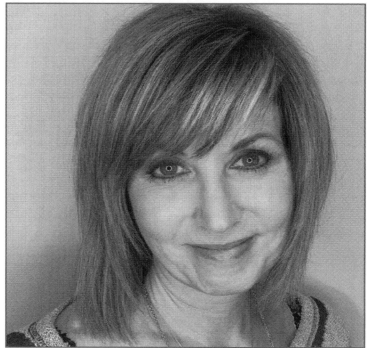

Lobs are bobs with extra length, and women who aren't ready to go too short appreciate them as a transitional style. If you currently have medium-length hair, all you need to do is cut a few inches off and request a razored finish to avoid bulky ends. Front bangs may provide a whimsical, youthful touch.

MARGARET R. SAXTON

Wavy Shaggy Copper Blonde Bob

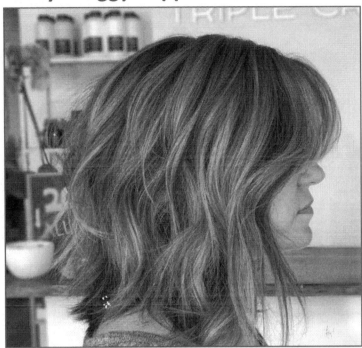

You are really fortunate if you are a lady over 50 with extremely thick hair! Allow your hair to graze your shoulders to show off your joy. Use natural-looking ocean waves to frame your face and highlight your best features. Balayage in caramel and honey complements the majority of complexion tones.

Feathered Blonde Balayage Pixie

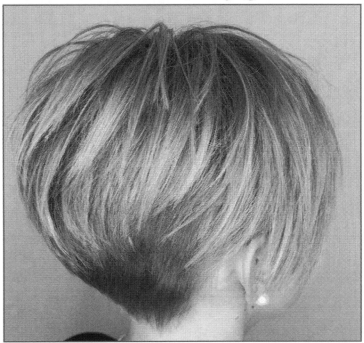

For women who are always on the move, worrying over hair style is just another source of stress. You'll have a style that's ready to go at any time with this stacked pixie cut for thin hair. The feathery layers give the cut a pleasing shape and provide volume, resulting in less labor for you.

Over 50 Shorter Feathered Blonde Hairstyle

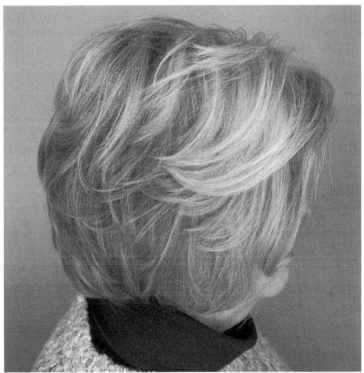

To raise your face and neckline, try a charming feathery chin-length bob. The wavy locks make the haircut fresh and lively, but if you want a "tamer" look, blow-dry it into a classic bob and tuck the sides behind your ears.

MARGARET R. SAXTON

Over 50 Feathered Silver Pixie with Bangs

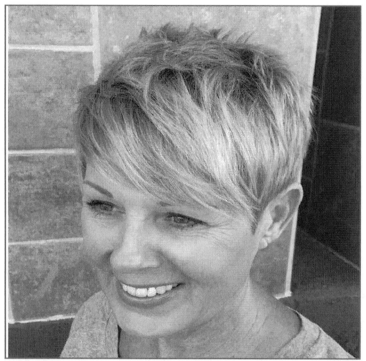

When deciding on the best pixie cut for you, check through photographs of trendy styles and consider how much time you want to spend on styling. Try a textured cut with medium layers and a short back if you just have a few minutes to primp in the morning.

Mid-Length Feathered Beige Blonde Hairstyle

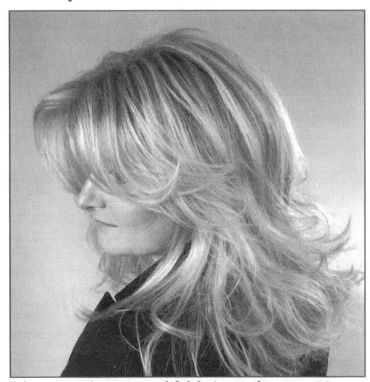

When you choose youthful haircuts for over 50, you run the danger of seeming like you're trying too hard to be young. This isn't the case with this mid-length shaggy style. It flatteringly frames the face and neck, and the soft golden balayage takes it to the next level of refinement.

MARGARET R. SAXTON

62

Short-to-Medium Hairstyle with Layers

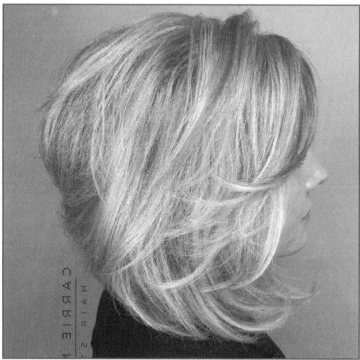

Consider the in-between phase of a cut. If you want a cropped look but aren't ready to commit to a pixie, try a collarbone cut. With some swooping layers, you'll never feel like you're wearing an odd mid length.

Medium-Length Golden Bob

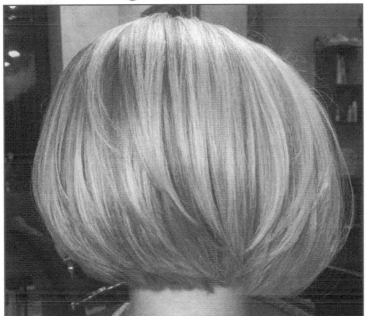

Most people believe that hairstyles for women over 50 must forgo length and color. Thankfully, they're mistaken, as seen by this beautiful blonde bob. Blonde highlights on a honey blonde foundation coupled with a sleek, voluminous haircut creates a glamorous and elegant look that is appropriate for women of all ages.

Reverse-Ombre for Short Gray Hair

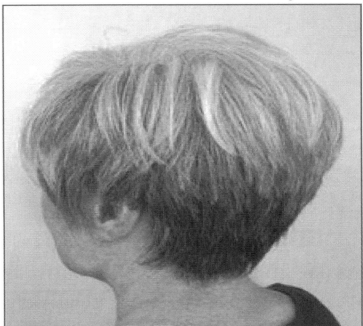

Traditional ombre techniques begin dark at the roots and fade lighter towards the ends, but fading from light to dark not only offers an overall brighter appearance, but also adds amazing depth. This color combination is ideal for individuals who do not want to go gray all over, since the black contrast keeps a young edge.

Short Piece-y Crop

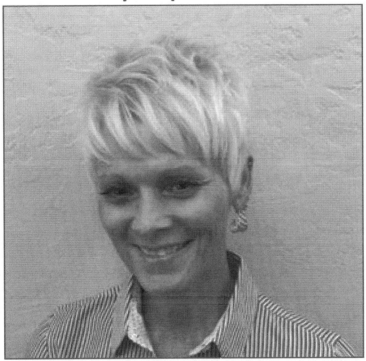

A sleek crop is lovely, but a pieced-together crop may be just as stylish. To add texture and define the ends of your layers, use a little style gel or mousse. This will assist you in creating a truly awesome, edgy style.

Neat Feathered Gray Pixie

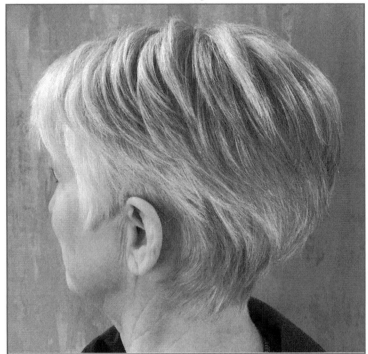

A nice pixie cut is a timeless option for middle-aged ladies looking for a change. It needs the least upkeep and is the perfect "wake up and go" look - what could be simpler? For a nice and clean form, choose for somewhat longer strands on top and around the face, but keep hair tightly trimmed towards the nape of the neck.

Choppy Bronde Pixie

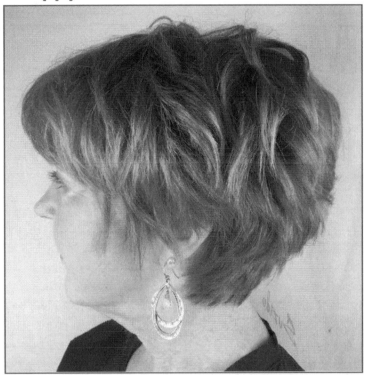

One of the greatest haircut styles for women over 50 who wish to keep their hair trimmed is the classic pixie. If your hair is thick, choose choppy layers to keep it from seeming poufy and uncontrolled.

Medium Thick Feathered Cut

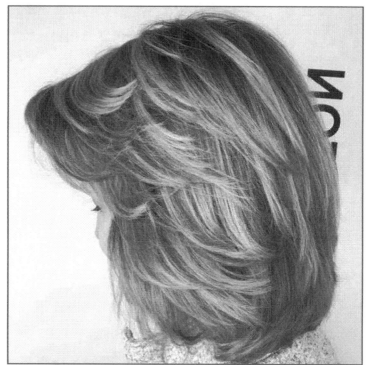

The honey-toned feathery cut is a lovely way to show off your healthy, thick hair. The layers provide movement to the hairdo, making it thick and dense yet not blocky.

Lob with Swoopy Bangs for Thick Hair

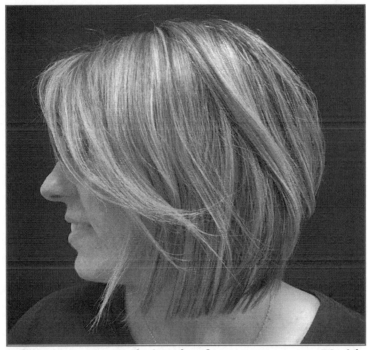

When it comes to hairstyles for women over 50, it's critical to choose something that won't seem antiquated. A highly sleek and straight bob, especially when well-maintained, always feels current and stylish. Make a rounder bottom with big curlers and finish with nourishing oil for added shine.

MARGARET R. SAXTON

Medium Hair with Sweeping Layers

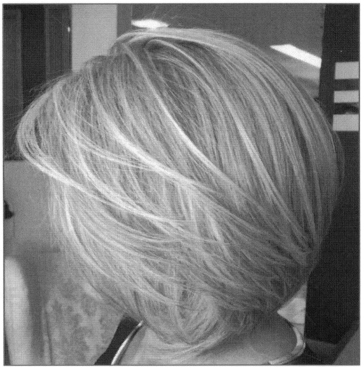

There's nothing wrong with an air-dried 'do, but a brush-styled 'do always has a refined finish. These layers are lightly swept away from the face to add movement.

Medium Layered Haircut

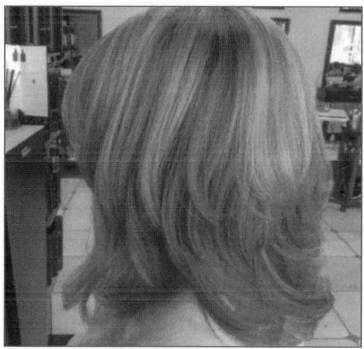

This gorgeous cut with gentle layers and honey highlights looks wonderful on pale skin tones. To get the seamless look, your longest locks should reach your shoulders, while the top layers are gradually chopped shorter. Aside from looking wonderful, the hairstyle is also pretty simple to maintain - finish the look with side-swept bangs on the front and shape the tips with a round brush.

MARGARET R. SAXTON

Long Choppy Bob with Bangs for Women Over 50

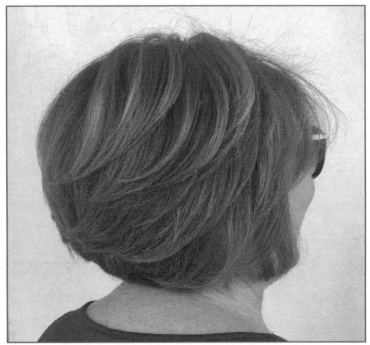

50-year-olds frequently cut their hair short since maintaining long locks is difficult and does not always appear age-appropriate. If you don't want to change the length of your hair, an a-line lob is a great option: the back will open up the neckline while your face-framing layers will still skim your shoulders up front.

Blonde Cropped Hairstyle

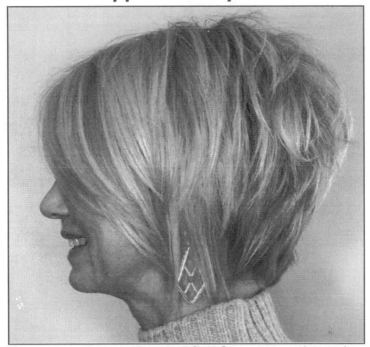

The appropriate cut is appealing from every viewpoint. You don't always notice your style from the rear, but others do. A fuller head of hair is created by a style that smoothly tapers towards the neck through feathery layers.

Medium Blonde Balayage Hairstyle with Dynamic Layers

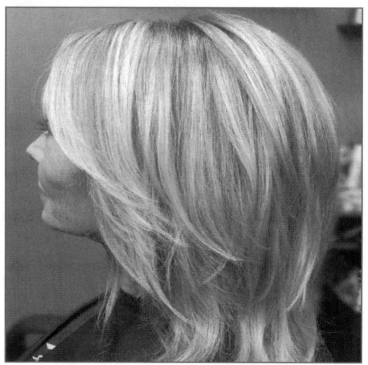

Just because you're in your forties doesn't mean you can't have fun with your haircut! When you're 50 and over, there's a lot you can do with medium hairstyles, so experiment with fresh highlights and sassy layers. You're never too old to add some zing to your look!

MARGARET R. SAXTON

Shorter Feathered Red and Blonde Hairstyle

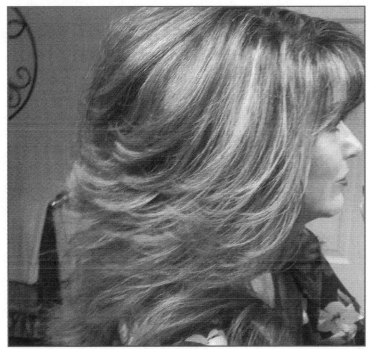

A red and blonde color combination isn't easy to pull off, but when you do, the outcome is stunning. Medium hairstyles with longer layers that feather in a sweeping motion look best with this two-toned hue because it provides dimension and helps you to truly show off the subtleties of the form.

Soft Curly Blonde Bob

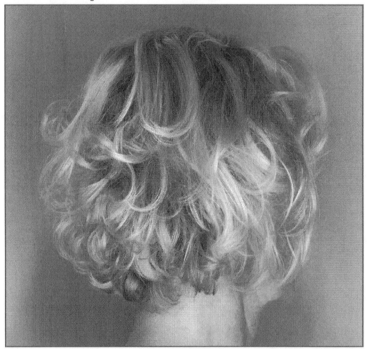

Choose a style that emphasizes your hair's natural texture. Women with curly or wavy hair might benefit from a deva cut, which allows for a smooth wash-and-go hairdo that makes your curls sparkle.

Brown Blonde Layered Hairstyle

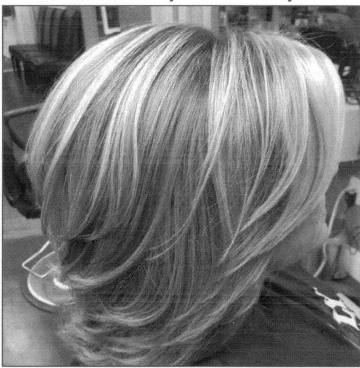

Take a look at how these layers fall. It appears to be a difficult 'do to style at home, but it isn't. Request that your hairdresser create feathery layers in your hair. Use a round brush to flick the ends of your hair towards the back while blow drying it. Apply hairspray to finish.

Hairstyle with Feathery Layers and Nape Undercut

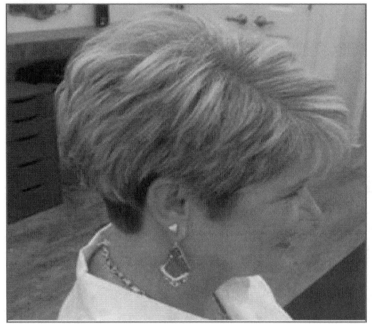

Keeping hair short and neat may be a very useful option for older ladies who are weary of maintaining longer locks. To keep some volume, trim stacked and feathered layers and match them with beautiful side bangs.

Medium White Blonde Feathered Hairstyle

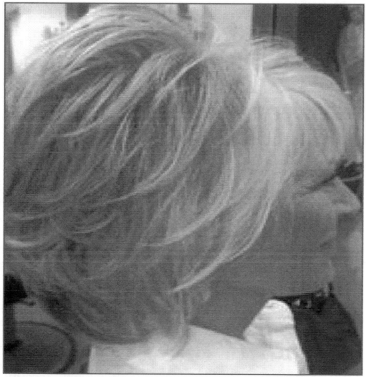

Layers carefully trimmed can change medium-to-short hairstyles for women over 50. If you have fine, thin hair, feathery layers are a fantastic method to add volume and lift to your mane. This low-maintenance style is popular among girls over 50. It helps you preserve your youthful radiance.

MARGARET R. SAXTON

50+ Short Curly Salt and Pepper Bob

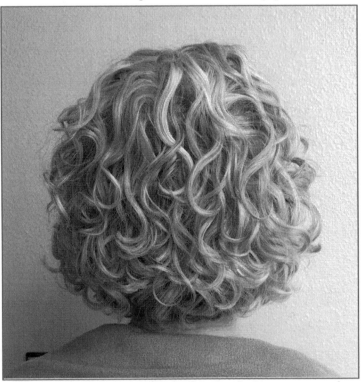

Finding a look that works with your hair texture rather than against it is the key to perfecting hairstyles for women with thick hair. When hair is finely curled, it holds its shape well, which is why a bob might be a good choice. Brush short, curly hair when it's damp, as dry brushing might result in an excessively fluffy finish.

Blonde Feathered Bob with Height on the Crown

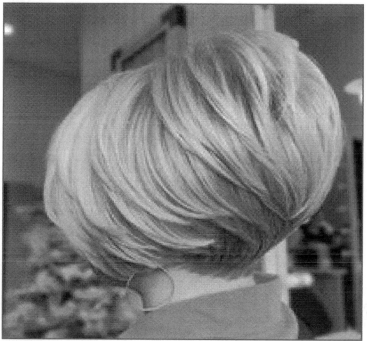

Feathered layers are playful and delightful, especially when teased in the back to elevate the crown. Request chin-length layers in the front that become shorter and shorter towards the rear, as well as some long bangs from your hairdresser. To style, blow dry with a round brush, tease the back, and you're ready to go.

MARGARET R. SAXTON

Medium Layered Hairstyle with Bangs

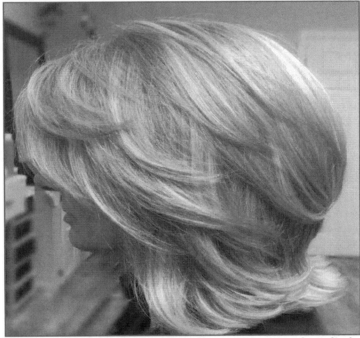

Today, most hairdressers believe that age has little bearing on haircut choices. You may choose any haircut that looks well on your face, hair type, and personality. However, on women in their 50s, fairly voluminous short and medium hairstyles appear better than smooth ones. This layered look with delicate accents is stunning.

MARGARET R. SAXTON

Short Auburn Bob with Layers

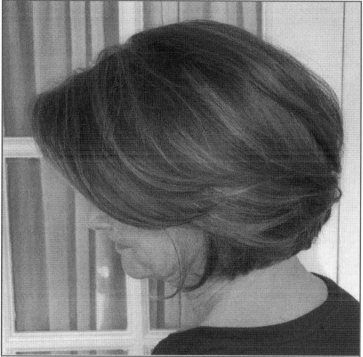

If you choose a layered bob, make sure it is styled to highlight your dynamic cut. The way these shorter layers have been combed back and set results in a cool take on feathered hair.

Bob with Flicked Ends

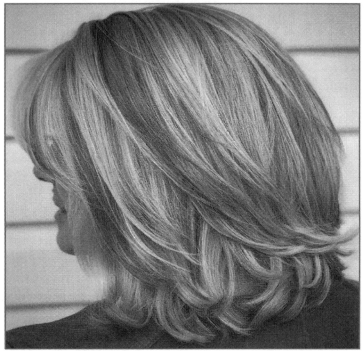

Today's hairstyles for women over 50 make it simple to incorporate your natural grays into contemporary color jobs. To blend gray with deeper blondes or browns, use the balayage process. Cut lengthy layers into your hairstyle to create delicate movement.

MARGARET R. SAXTON

Made in the USA
Las Vegas, NV
30 September 2023

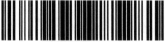

78345042R00048